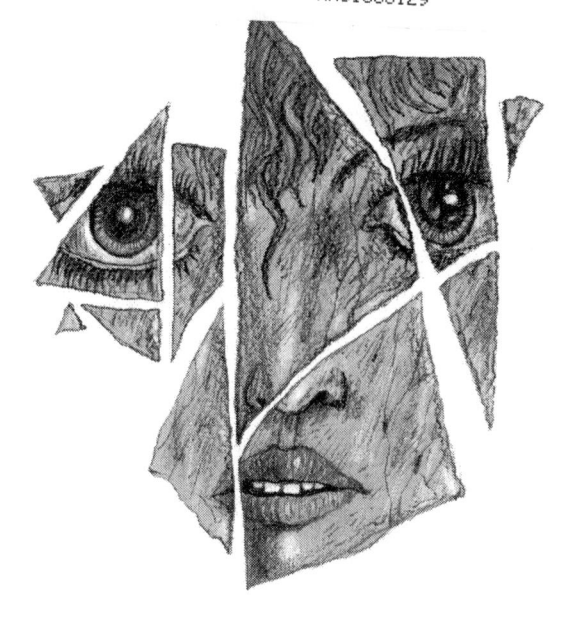

# UNCOMMON COURAGE

Faith, Hope and Love
support a mother and daughter
when schizophrenia shatters their world

Cheryl Wiker

# UNCOMMON COURAGE

*Faith, Hope and Love support a mother and daughter when schizophrenia shatters their world*

*This book is dedicated to my wonderful husband,*
*Rick Wiker.*
*There are no words to express my gratitude for a lifetime of*
*love and support for our children.*

# Table of Contents

# Introduction

Many years have passed since I lost my daughter Kim. Her death was not physical although many times I wished she might have been lost to us like that. Death is often merciful as we realize our loved one no longer suffers.

But the disintegration of a brain which was once rational and vibrant creates a lifetime of emotional pain and stress for families as they attempt to cope with hallucinations and bizarre behaviors that afflict their child seemingly overnight.

Kim was a typical 16-year-old when schizophrenia took her from us. This tragic disease disables 1.5 million people in the world each year. The lives of these sufferers will bring constant worry, anxiety and deep sorrow to their families. Their parents will begin the stressful education about an illness they probably never even contemplated, until their beloved child was slammed with it like a semi-truck head on collision.

I decided to write our story because we can all find inspiration in Kim's uncommon courage which inspires her to find meaning in life, despite a brain that often seems to be her greatest enemy.

Kim's story makes it crystal clear that **faith, hope and love** allow us to survive every storm, and even smile with genuine joy and gratitude. *The main goal of this book is to remind us to rely on faith, hope and love when facing any challenge that has the power to make us or break us. We can find strength for another day if we* **rely on even one of these powerful spiritual energies.**

This is a short book because the people who need it the most are those who are dealing with pain and loss. If you are experiencing an emotional tsunami, you probably don't have the energy to wade through a long book.

Faith can be experienced in many forms. Sometimes we have faith in our own ability and when that isn't enough, we can rely on faith in a higher power. It is also empowering as we learn to trust or put our faith in friends, family and our community.

Our story also reminds us that we are never alone in our struggle if we are willing to ask for help. Social workers, psychiatrists, and volunteers who give generously of their time and energy, are often the reason patients and families can make it through their week.

Despite their reputations, there are many attorneys who have huge hearts and serve the community with integrity and genuine concern. They provided invaluable aid when Kim was missing from the San Antonio State Hospital for three terrifying days.

Hopefully some politicians will also be moved to increase funding for support systems which care for our mentally ill. My brother told me a horrifying story about his experience as a policeman in the Washington DC suburbs. The budget for the mentally ill was slashed and St. Elizabeth's hospital in Washington DC, simply released many mentally ill patients. Local police were continuously called to assist those left homeless and adrift. Their "assistance" meant a trip to the police station and brief incarceration! This was not just one or two patients.

There were hundreds of them, and the police could not focus on real crime when they were collecting the mentally ill, whose bizarre behavior frightened other citizens.

How can this happen?

Federal grants have been given for research that seems far less important than funding for our mentally ill. The following example is only one out of hundreds that reveal outrageous government waste.

The Pentagon was criticized in June 2017 for spending $28 million on licensing fees for the lush green pattern on Afghan National Army uniforms. The problem: Afghanistan is 98% desert, so the bright color would stand out- not what you're looking for in camouflage.

It's time to insist our politicians decrease wasteful spending and increase funding for our vulnerable mentally ill citizens.

We eventually moved to Michigan from Texas which was a God send for Kim. Michigan is superior when it comes to support for people with a mental health condition.

I took twenty-five years to share this story because my grief had to be put into perspective. Kim's life today is comfortable and stable. She will never be able to work or drive, but her spirit is joyful.

If asked, "Would you rather have died than have schizophrenia?" her response would be "I choose life!

*Life does not
have to be perfect
to be wonderful!*

# What just happened?

Single parenting is always challenging but I preferred that challenge to its alternative. I found my marriage suffocating because I deeply desired to explore different spiritual perspectives.

My three children grew up in a rigid, strict religious home that allowed no normal testing of limits by children. An atmosphere of fear permeated our home since any breach of boundaries was met with severe punishment. We all learned to stay in line in order to have some peace.

As my children approached their teen years, I knew they would never be allowed to break away from their parents and develop their own ideas and beliefs. The decision to divorce was made after waking up in the middle of the night with tears soaking my pillow.

I had started to lay a financial foundation a year before filing. Teaching piano created an independent income which also allowed me to work from home. I never experienced the grief many people have after a divorce. I felt relief and great joy, in my rediscovered freedom to grow and expand. I gave this same freedom to my children, Kim, Rachele and Keith. I told them there was only one rule in the house now. They must never to do anything that would hurt themselves or others.

My son had deep anxiety which manifested through bed wetting. After his father moved out, he never wet the bed again. He was 11 years old so that was all the validation I needed to know the divorce was in their highest and best interest.

I also had a dream one night that gave me the strength and faith to free myself. In the dream, I heard God telling me that He would provide for us. My husband had been the financial provider, but I saw God's love was our real Source of security.

As months passed, I was able to pay bills on time, and my faith turned into confidence that all would be well. Little did I know that a storm was coming that would require every ounce of faith and strength to endure.

"Mom, be quiet." Kim and I were silently eating dinner on TV trays one evening. Her statement startled me.

"I didn't say anything!" I responded. I didn't think much of it until a few minutes later.

"I told you to stop saying that!" she exclaimed.

This time I was alarmed. "What do you think I am saying honey? I really have not said a word!"

"I can hear you!" she responded. "You are telling me I am ugly, and you hate me!"

This is probably the first and only time I was genuinely stunned in my life.

"Kim, I would NEVER say something like that. That's awful! Why would you say that?"

She did not respond but stared vacantly at the TV. I was not sure what to do next so prayed for guidance.

The next thing that came out of her mouth brought me out of prayer and into action.

"If you don't stop saying that I am going to get a baseball bat."

She thought I was telling her I hated her and was going to hurt her. I realized her comment about the baseball bat was not just an idle threat. It terrified me but the waves of fear pushed me into action. I went to my bedroom and locked the door. I called Helen, a friend from church who was also the nurse at the High School Kim attended.

Helen immediately said, "Cheryl, this sounds like paranoid schizophrenia. You need to get her to a doctor right away."

I barely slept that night. I was relieved when she finally went to sleep, but I checked on her throughout the night. I was aware something scary was taking place in her mind, but I was also afraid for her sister and brother who were sleeping close by. I can only imagine the anxiety they must have felt, wondering what was happening to their older sister.

Fortunately, her dad was still in town and not traveling with his missionary trips. He was as concerned as I was when he received my call. He could be hard to deal with at times, but I knew he loved the children. He just wasn't equipped emotionally to express warmth and compassion.

The very next morning we took her to the hospital, unaware that she would not be home for a very, very long time.

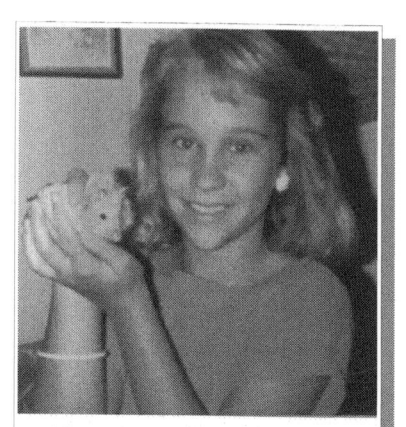

Kim enjoys a normal childhood
at 14 years old—two years before
the onset of schizophrenia

# No end in sight

There are usually some symptoms displayed before the actual psychotic break. Unfortunately, many of these could merely be teenage hormones kicking into high gear. I thought I was tuned in to my children but as a single parent focused on working enough to provide for their physical needs, I missed some of these telltale signs.

One of Kim's friends had been worried about her. Kim had always been sociable, but she had been sitting by herself for lunch every day for several months. *Big red flag!* She had also demonstrated some uncharacteristic violent behavior toward he sister, Rachele. They shared a room and quarrels were frequent with any breach of boundaries. One source of friction was the jealousy that Kim experienced with babysitting jobs.

As the girls became teenagers, Kim was often asked to babysit other children in the apartment complex. She was older than Rachele, so people thought of her first when looking for a babysitter. If she could not do it for some reason, Rachele would offer to help. Every time this happened, the parents always asked for Rachele after her first time with their children. I felt bad for Kim, because Rachele had the sweeter temperament and much more patience with the children. Naturally Kim felt the sting of rejection every time this happened.

However, I was not prepared for the day I heard a loud crash in their bedroom. Kim was enraged about something and she pulled over a heavy bookshelf, breaking it to pieces. This was the catalyst for moving her bed to the living room. I had no way of knowing that this violent outburst was a precursor to a much more devastating illness. I remembered it vividly though, when she forcefully said she was going to get a baseball bat!

Colonial Hills was a private psychiatric hospital in San Antonio, Texas. Kim was admitted for evaluation since her delusions were so extreme. My heart sank when we met with the doctor at the end of her two weeks stay in the private hospital. That was the limit on the bed she now occupied as a charity case because we did not have medical insurance.

The doctor gently informed us, "Kim needs much more treatment than we can give her here. Since there is no insurance, we need to transfer her to the adolescent unit at the state hospital in San Antonio."

I tried to hug her, but she was descending deeper into psychosis and was very paranoid. Paranoid schizophrenia is scary for all involved. The sufferers are convinced that others want to hurt them, and they can become very aggressive in their self-defense. A dear friend told me the heartbreaking story of losing his best friend as a result of paranoid schizophrenia. His friend Bill was in his late seventies and somewhat frail. Bill's daughter suffered with this illness. He had cared for her often and felt secure enough to take a nap one day when she was visiting his home. He woke up to the horrifying realization that he was being stabbed to death by his daughter!

This story made me realize I would always need to keep a degree of vigilance and caution, even when Kim appeared stable. But at the time I was still trying to come to grips with how much life was changing for Kim and our family.

I went into culture shock as my world expanded when I encountered the San Antonio State Hospital for the first time. Sometimes our world is enlarged as we see the bigger picture. My bigger picture looked more like a distorted abstract painting. This was a whole new and frightening world right on the doorstep that I was totally unaware of, until Kim became part of it.

There was nothing homey or cozy about this institution for the mentally ill. Patients slumped in chairs or wandered around aimlessly, shuffling in their hospital issued slippers. The adolescent unit had none of the teenage vitality you might expect or imagine. Heavy sedation made them easier to manage.

Her memories of the time there are truly sad. Patients were not allowed to watch much TV, which I imagine was to avoid arguing or fighting over what shows to watch. Kim learned to swear and hit back while there. She never heard vulgar language in our home, so it was unsettling to hear the profanity that popped out with ease now.

Two girls, Jennifer and Tracy, were particularly mean. When Jennifer gave Kim a menacing look, Kim's paranoia motivated her to tell a staff member. Jennifer followed up by grabbing Kim by the neck and bashing her head into the ping pong table.

Tracy was only 15 but a real bully according to Kim. She was constantly unkind and one day hit her for no reason. Kim decided enough was enough and hit back. Tracy took her down and smashed her head into the floor. The girl was a street hardened gang member with fighting experience. She spent her long boring days looking for new ways to harass the more vulnerable patients. Kim was easy prey and no match for her. This time the staff stepped in and put both girls in a time out room for hours. Kim's head was bleeding, and she cried herself to sleep.

The most heartbreaking memory for me was her simple statement: "I mostly sat alone, wishing I could go home."

We lived in New Braunfels which was a fifty-minute drive to the San Antonio State hospital. Life now included a weekly trip to the hospital to see Kim. I desperately wanted to see her more often, but I still had two other children who needed a secure home. They needed my presence and attention also. Since my divorce, I had full time custody because their dad often traveled with his job. Many people think their job creates stress, but for me work was a relief from stress because I could focus on something other than Kim's suffering.

One particularly discouraging visit to the hospital reduced me to an emotional basket case. That weekend was a traumatic one for Kim and as soon as I entered the room, she jumped onto the bed screaming, "I hate you! Get away from me! You are the devil! Stay away." She stayed on her bed to protect herself from the devil she thought I had become. No amount of talking could get her to calm down and they took her away to a room where they strapped patients down. This was called "four pointing" the patient.

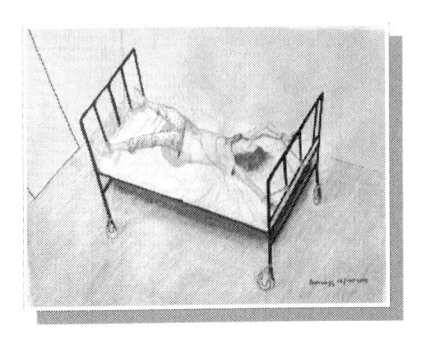

Visiting her each week became a heart wrenching experience. I always came intending to smile and bring as much love as I could, only to be reduced to a puddle of anguish and tears at the end of the visit. Her psychotic delusions often made it impossible to carry on a conversation and I simply hoped she could remember family had visited that week.

Her father also visited, and I worried about him too. We had always been very proud of Kim's bright mind and her love of learning. Kim was an avid reader. I will never forget how amazed I was when I found her reading an animal story in the Readers Digest at six years old! I even quizzed her comprehension and realized she understood everything she was reading. We had high hopes for her life.

After the first year in the adolescent unit, she was stable enough to attend the high school classes the hospital offered. There were only five teens in her class, but it was a positive step that gave me hope she might improve enough to come home. I will let Kim share some of her memories with you.

*"I remember seeing some kids getting into a line by the door of our unit. I decided to get in line with them and nobody stopped me! I followed them to the school building and pretended I belonged there. Later, they asked me if I wanted to go to school. I really enjoyed having something to do and went for half a day on school days. We studied science, English and they even let us play games on the computers. I wrote lots of poems, but the voices made me tear them up. I got a high school diploma, but the voices made me tear it up too."*

This progress led to a new level of advancement. The doctors decided to see how she would do in the transitional care unit which was designed to prepare patients to live outside of the hospital. However, her progress was short lived. After the doctors had used every medication available to them, I was called in for a meeting. The doctor's words held no hope. "We are transferring Kim to the long-term care unit next week. We think we can give her better extended care there."

At some point I quit trying to figure out what went wrong. Nothing made sense when her brain was so bizarre. The doctors had no insights either. I wondered why anyone would want to spend their life trying to work with mentally ill people, knowing their patients would never be cured.

The doctors put patients in the long-term care unit when they have no real hope of improvement. I saw the patients in this unit. Many were older people who had been there for twenty or thirty years. Visiting this unit tore my heart out. There were no young people and the geriatric patients were physically and mentally feeble. The building even smelled old and musty. I could not imagine young Kim spending her life in this hopelessly sad place. I had to sit down before my legs collapsed from the grief that now overpowered me.

On the drive home I had to pull off the road because the pain and tears made driving impossible. I wished God had taken Kim to heaven so she would be free of suffering. My heart began to physically hurt because of the unrelenting emotional pain. Waves of pure pulsating pain overwhelmed me.

Mental health workers told me that many family members no longer visit patients because they cannot cope with this emotional pain. It isn't a lack of love. It is impossible to live any kind of life in this emotional torture chamber. As I sat by the road trying to cry it out, I kept holding my chest because the pain sent an aching throb that was as much physical as emotional. The reality of the situation hit home because I realized people were not made to live with this kind of sustained pain. I thought I might be having a heart attack.

I could not drive, and an illuminating thought seemed to come from out of the blue. I became aware that I was getting help from a much higher power. It said, "From this day forward you must begin to express gratitude for everything in Kim's life. This is the only way you are going to survive this."

The thought was powerful, however, I wondered what I could be grateful for since she didn't appear to have a life anymore. But the survival instinct kicked in and I began to thank God for every little thing that I could imagine.

"Thank you for clean sheets she sleeps on every night. Thank you for the three meals a day someone prepares for her. Thank you for the fresh air she breathes. Thank you for the family that loves her. Thank you for the doctors and staff that care for her every day. Thank you for anyone that shares a moment of kindness in her day." I even thanked God for her good teeth! I noticed my heart was beginning to calm down and a new peace came to my soul. I thanked God for His love for Kim. The pain did not vanish, but it became manageable. This became my reality for several years.

Just when I thought things could not get worse, I discovered there was a deeper dimension to hell on earth. It would lead to a three-year court case and trial by jury!

# Letting go of all hope

There are no straight roads on the journey through schizophrenia. Just when new hope is on the horizon, it is often sabotaged by the setbacks most sufferers experience. Before I was informed of the hospital decision to transfer Kim to the long-term care unit, I had hope that she might be home soon.

The patients had levels assigned that extended privileges based upon their behavior. Kim had stabilized enough that she was able to wear her own clothes and go outside on unsupervised walks around the hospital grounds. This was a level four privilege that also allowed her to work in the thrift shop and do laundry. She still remembers ironing the underwear with laundry duty!

This was a vast improvement from her memories of being beaten up and "four pointed" to the bed. She has scars on her knuckles from hitting the wall when put in the time out room for hours at a time. When asked what she remembers about the other five students in the high school classes she attended, she surprised me with her response. "Mom, some of them were real gangsters! They had gang tattoos on their arms and faces." Kim had grown up surrounded by church friends and wholesome school friends. This world was a huge culture shock for her.

I was thrilled when she was considered for the transitional living facility. This was still on the hospital grounds, but it was a huge step forward with the goal of preparing for the world outside of the institutional routines. She now shared a private room with a single roommate which was quite a treat since there were ten beds per room in adolescent building. Each room had a private bath with a vanity, and she had her own key to her locked closet. This small amount of privacy was now a luxury she enjoyed tremendously. However, Kim's fondest memory is how good the food was, and they could even have seconds if they wanted it!

One of the exercises to prepare them for living outside the hospital was to apply for a job somewhere off the hospital grounds. Kim was in the hospital van with some other patients and staff. She was hoping to apply for a job at the Marriott hotel. As they passed through the gate, the attendant asked to see her green pass which verified authorization to leave the hospital. For some reason this created a stress reaction from Kim that immediately dropped her from a level 4 to a 1.

We will never understand what caused another psychotic break. When asked what really happened, she says, "Mom, they arrested me just because I used the "B" word with that rude lady!" She was quickly transferred to the long-term care unit.

Her worst nightmare was about to come to life. I am thankful at times that we cannot see the future. Living one day at a time is not just a nice spiritual concept. It is how families survive when in crisis.

# Funny friends are the best therapy!

I could never bring myself to attend the support groups for schizophrenia. Dealing with my own pain was all I could handle. Sharing the pain with a roomful of other suffering families was overwhelming and draining. I found another way to numb the pain.

Everyone should have a friend like Toby Skroder. Having fun with Toby made life bearable as we created many ways to laugh. My sadness was often bearable because of the silly things we did to bring some much-needed fun to life. Toby was a dance instructor with a studio in a three-story building. The second story had a room containing hundreds of rubber duckies that were floated down the San Antonio River walk once a year. We decided it was a fine idea to borrow the rubber duckies to decorate the front yard of my very serious straight-laced pastor. He was a wonderful churchman, but we thought he could use some lightening up.

We went to great lengths to find new ways to laugh instead of cry. I love life and fought hard to find some joy amid the pain. If joy could not be found, then we would create it! Our greatest source of silliness was the creation of the Succotash Sisters, Maybelle and Emmy Lou. For some reason we thought it would be fun to create our own comic characters who performed without a stage.

Maybelle and Emmy Lou spoke with an exaggerated hillbilly drawl and were always coming up with ways to entertain people. In truth, Toby and I probably laughed much harder at ourselves than others did, but we didn't care. One year the Succotash Sisters made a pin up calendar for Toby's husband, John, featuring Maybelle and Emmylou antics from selling outhouse real-estate to fun in the sun swimming for the month of June. It remains one of my favorite lifetime memories.

The Succotash Sisters keep us laughing
instead of crying

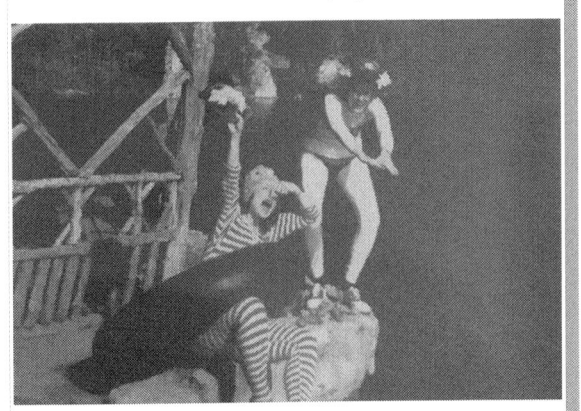

*"When M & E come with ther beech atire,
all the men's harts gits loaded with FIRE!"*

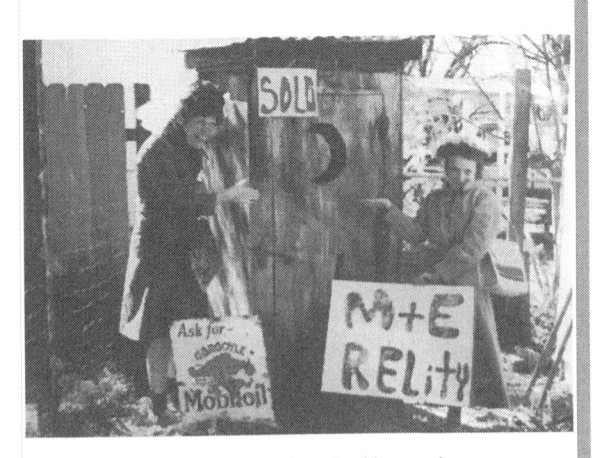

*"Life ain't jest a bunch o' horseplay.
You whould work if yur strong n' able.
Maybelle & Emmylous Relity puts vittles on ther table."*

So of course, Toby was the first person I called when a phone call came from the hospital that began three days of sheer agony. Toby was also a good shoulder to cry on.

"Mrs. Koehler, we need to speak with you right away. Kim is missing. We have scoured the hospital compound and she is not here." Panic and stomach-churning fear is the only response when your child is missing. Every fear imaginable runs through your mind. There is no relief, no pill, no advice or suggestion to calm the fear.

Faith and prayer became my lifeline to hope. I forced myself to trust (*faith*) she would be found. I *hoped* she was alive. *Love* energized me to find her.

# Who's in charge here!

I called Toby and we rushed to the hospital. We were informed Kim had left by a hole in the fence surrounding the compound. Toby and I went to the perimeter and stared with disbelief at the sizable hole with a mattress on the ground right next to it. Apparently, this was a well-known escape hatch for patients that the hospital knew about. Patients could simply leave the hospital any time they pleased!

How was it possible for court committed patients to leave the grounds whenever they wanted, to roam the streets of San Antonio? Court-committed patients were considered a danger to themselves or others. To make it even more incomprehensible, the hospital's official visitors gate was within sight of this hole in the fence. The gate had an attendant who checked the passes which authorized entrance. Many questions needed answering, but my immediate priority was to try and find Kim in a city of 1.5 *million* people!

My stomach was often queasy as fear created worst case scenarios in my imagination. Kim was so naïve! How would she survive on the streets with her delusions and total lack of street smarts? Worse, she would suddenly be off her medication which was very scary. She was at serious risk for feeling sick physically and having even worse hallucinations. Kim was tormented by aural hallucinations. The voices in her head were not just "thoughts". They were very real voices that commanded her to do things. She thought it was the voice of God and she would obey without question.

I returned to the hospital's administrative office to find out what they were doing to find her. They viewed me as an adversary now when I asked about this hole in the fence that seemed to be common knowledge. They said the San Antonio Police department had been informed and her situation was now out of their hands. The police department was my next stop and I couldn't believe my ears when they said there was a full-time officer assigned to collect missing patients from the State Hospital! My mind was begging, *"What's wrong with this picture?"*

Later that day the hospital let me know they had some information which could be helpful. "We have spoken to some of the patients and they believe Kim was taken out by a man who was once a patient at the hospital." His name was Raul Chapa. A social worker at the hospital confided in me: "Mr. Chapa is a sociopath whose legal offenses had landed him in the State Hospital instead of jail."

The definition of a sociopath is "a mental health condition in which a person has a long-term pattern of manipulating, exploiting, or violating the rights of others." I now had no hope that some kind stranger would realize Kim needed help and return her to safety.

For three agonizing days I drove the streets within walking distance of the hospital, desperate to get a glimpse of her. Hoping her bizarre behavior might have made her memorable, I showed her picture to hundreds of shop employees and anyone passing by that was willing to stop for a moment.

"Have you seen my daughter?", was met with sympathy but nobody remembered her.

The fourth morning a call finally came from the hospital, "Kim was found by the police and she is at the medical hospital for examination." A rape counselor was with Kim when I arrived, and I struggled to hold back the tears as Kim told us of her nightmare. I also realized she was lucky to be alive.

Raul had given her a ring and told her they were now married. At some point in the three days she was locked in a room at a boarding house where he repeatedly raped her. When she resisted, he insisted they were married, and she had to have sex with him.

On the third day as he approached her again, she grabbed a belt and started swinging it to defend herself. He grabbed it and threw her to the ground as she kicked and screamed for help. Fortunately, a man from another room came to her rescue, after hearing her screams. She gratefully accepted refuge in this stranger's room and fell asleep, only to be awakened by Mr. Chapa rampaging with a knife as he tried to break in to get her back. She somehow escaped the room and pounded on the door to another room. Thankfully the occupant let her in, and the police were finally called.

It's almost impossible to describe the layers of anger and pain I experienced, trying to comprehend what she had just experienced. Kim was a virgin, and this was her first sexual experience. What should have been a wonderful memory with someone she loved would now be her worst memory for life, filled with fear, anguish and pain. This unforgivable situation challenged everything I had been taught about forgiveness. Sermons about forgiveness seemed shallow and powerless to heal the pain.

After Kim was back in the State hospital, I went to the police department to file charges. Raul Chapa needed to be arrested and removed from the streets of San Antonio! The police response shocked me completely: "You can certainly press charges, but you need to understand what will happen if you do. Mr. Chapa has a history of mental illness so he will never be sent to jail. He will be sent back to the State Hospital as a patient, and Kim will be more accessible to him there."

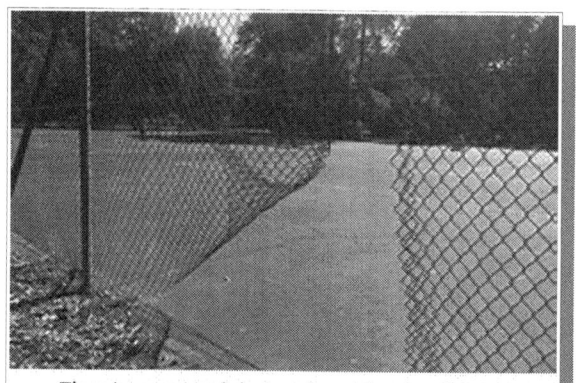

The pictures used during the trial are no longer available. This tear closely resembles some of the tears in the fence surrounding the San Antonio State Hospital at the time.

The decision to not press charges was only tolerable since Kim would be vulnerable if Raul was back at the hospital as a patient. He would never suffer any consequences for his crime but protecting Kim was my main goal and concern.

Oh, dear God, when would this nightmare end? At this point my pain gave birth to a burning anger over Kim's total lack of protection from the hospital. I decided it was time to find out who was in charge and hold them accountable for repairing and securing that fence. The court committed mentally ill patients deserved adequate protection and it seemed like such an easy thing to fix.

# An appointed time for everything

I never enjoyed being the center of attention. But it was time to be a squeaky wheel and get the hospital to fix the damn fence! Several visits to the hospital's administrative office led me to realize no one wanted to assume responsibility for this situation. Several times I was told to make a new appointment with someone who would "investigate" it further. These meetings made it obvious that they were never going to fix this problem.

At the time I was supplementing my teaching income with a part time job for a stock broker named Bill, who did a weekly stock report for KSAT 12 news in San Antonio. He had some valuable connections. "Bill, I am beside myself with worry. The hospital refuses to fix that fence and I know Kim is not safe there. And if she is not safe there, that means the other patients are not safe." I was about to ask him for a huge favor.

"Do you think you could use your connections at the TV station to get them to do a news story about this situation? I think that might be what it takes to get them to do the right thing."

"That's a great idea," Bill responded enthusiastically. And he was as good as his word.

Within days, Tony Fama, one of the station's top investigative reporters, had a camera crew in place to shed some much-needed light on the plight of the mentally ill at the hospital. They did an excellent job of sharing Kim's story and showing where she was easily abducted through the huge hole in the fence.

During the on-site filming, a hospital security van pulled up but did not say anything. They simply observed the situation to report back to their supervisors. The hospital administrators did nothing in response. I started to wonder if the patients were running the hospital!

One of the best things we can learn through the passage of time is to recognize there are reasons when a door doesn't open after repeatedly knocking. But I didn't have this wonderful insight at the time. What I did have was righteous anger building inside, fueled by constant concern for Kim's safety. In the 1990's we still used big bulky telephone books. I decided to use one to find an attorney to see if legal action would be possible. As a single parent I had no way to pay for representation but decided to act in blind faith and see what might happen. I never opened the phone book because right on the back cover was a full-page ad for one of the largest law firms in San Antonio: Branton & Hall. I called, and they were willing to make an appointment to talk with me. I prayed on the way to that meeting.

"God, please give me favor with these lawyers so Kim and the other patients can have better protection from the hospital."

The entrance to the firm was impressive and I was seated in a conference room to meet with Jim Hall. He was generous with his time and gracious, listening intently as I shared my story with him. I was aware that this was now in God's hands and I was doing everything I could possibly do to help my daughter and the other patients. In my mind and heart, Kim now represented all the other patients who didn't have families to fight for them. Mr. Hall's genuine caring and response had me singing on the way home. His law firm had decided to take the case on a contingency basis as a service to the community! Tom Crosley was assigned lead counsel for our law suit.

Later, I discovered they had been advised by colleagues from other firms not to do it. Suing the State was never profitable and there was a cap on the amount of money you could collect in damages. I didn't care about the money. I wanted the fence fixed. Surely the hospital would fix it quickly now that they faced a law suit.

A common cliché, "timing is everything" proved true in our case. Kim could have spent the rest of her life in the long-term care unit of the hospital if they had fixed the fence at that time! There was a medication that was unavailable to patients in the hospital. This medication would make her life much better or at least, far less tormented. But she would have to be released from the hospital to benefit from this new drug. Fixing the fence would calm my fears for her safety and I would have accepted the long-term care unit as our only option.

> *To everything there is a season & a time to every purpose under heaven.*
> *Ecclesiastes 3:1*

# Going home!

"The wheels of justice turn slowly" is frustratingly accurate. A typical negligence case can take a year or more to reach a verdict. However, a lawsuit involving the government will be much longer. Tom Crosley, lead counsel for the case, shared his summary of the trial. The hospital had the audacity to claim, *"the fence was not for security, and therefore, a hole in the fence did not pose an unreasonable risk of harm to the plaintiff."*

I wondered if the people who mounted this absurd defense would change their tune quickly if it had been their daughter wandering the streets of a large city with a sociopath. Would such empathy ever appear within the halls of justice? Anxiety over Kim's new situation began to erode my energy. How could I leave her in that hospital when that fence was not repaired? The hospital now refused to repair it because they defended their right to have holes in it!

Many parents of a mentally ill child give up legal guardianship when they realize they could be held legally liable if their child commits a crime. I had to make that horrible decision and Kim was now a ward of the state of Texas. I could not just march in and demand they let me take her home. However, the law suit might make them think twice about refusing. Bringing her home would present huge new challenges because she was still prone to bizarre behavior and hallucinations. But she was my daughter and nobody else on earth could love her like me.

The hospital had still not repaired the fence since that would be an admission of guilt which could be detrimental to their defense in the law suit! So, without having a clue about how to manage her at home, I went to the hospital with my request.

"I no longer feel Kim is safe in this hospital. I need to take her home." I used one of my favorite prayers again. I prayed for favor with the hospital doctors, if it was in Kim's highest and best interest to come home. It seemed obvious that this was the case, as I had lost all confidence that the administration had much common sense. Facing a lawsuit from one of San Antonio's largest law firms made them more reasonable. They must have wondered what would happen if she were to go missing again or be hurt in any other situation while in their custody. Kim was quickly released to my custody.

I asked Kim what she remembers about coming home after a year and a half in the hospital. She lights up with pure joy, exclaiming, *"It was like paradise! I was so happy!"* Thankfully, she was never aware of how stressful it would be for her brother and sister. She was so happy to be home and didn't complain when I had her sleeping on the couch instead of sharing a room with Rachele.

Rachele was two years younger than Kim and she was a gentle sweet spirit who always put others before herself. In high school she was a straight A student and first chair for the flute section in the school band. I was proud of her for that accomplishment. She did it with a second-hand flute. The band director had encouraged me to replace it with a better instrument, if she hoped to make first chair. My slim budget did not allow for a new instrument, but Rachele was a gifted musician and her little Bundy flute made sweet music because of her skill. She did hold first chair during her senior year and received a much-needed scholarship for her first two years of college at St. Mary's University in San Antonio.

Keith was four years younger than Kim and he was an easy-going, gentle soul who shared my sense of humor. He could always make me laugh with his subtle innuendos and light-hearted approach to problems. One time when his Dad had been especially harsh, he plopped on my bed and said with a serious but mischievous undertone, "Oh Cheryl, what are we going to do with that man?!" I laughed and laughed and knew this boy would be heart of my heart forever.

He was not home often after Kim came home. After school he worked setting pins in a bowling alley and his friends drew him outside whenever he had free time. I knew better than to ask Rachele and Keith if I should bring Kim home. After the divorce I was determined that home would always be the place where we could rest and recharge our batteries. Bringing Kim home was not going to be easy for any of us!

Rachele remembers me hiding all the knives and sharp objects before we went to bed. She says, "I was so scared of her erratic behavior that I popped the screen off my bedroom window and kept a stool by the window to escape quickly if she came at me." I also told her to put a chair against the door at night.

I remembered my prayer from the time of Kim's release from the hospital. I had to trust that having her home was in her highest and best interest and somehow, we would be protected. I desperately searched for a way to help Kim and have some semblance of normal life in this stressful situation.

Paranoid Schizophrenia knows no "normal." Families deal with deep sorrow behind closed doors in their own ways. Tears become a comforting release for the grief which is always present, even when pushed briefly into subconscious mind for sheer survival.

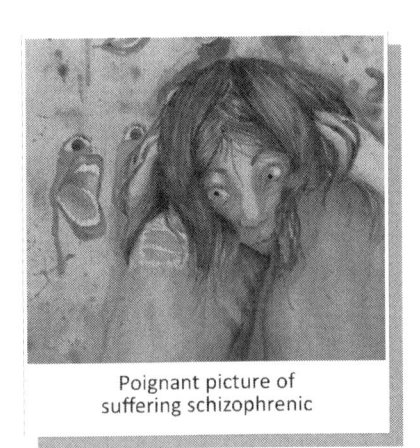

Poignant picture of
suffering schizophrenic

# Making the best of it

Keith and Rachele tried to make the best of it but their sister was not easy. Kim had always enjoyed bossing around her siblings, and she brought that tendency back into the household after her release from the hospital. Their way of coping was to hide out in their rooms. That didn't bother me much because I knew that most teens enjoy the privacy of their own rooms, even without a mentally ill sibling.

Home became a balancing act as I constantly tried to create a stable and peaceful environment. Working from home was another huge challenge. Fortunately, this 1200 square foot apartment had a huge master bedroom that allowed room for the piano. I screened off the bed and created the perfect little studio that even had access to the master bath for my piano students. This bedroom was immediately inside the entrance to the apartment, so my children still had a sense of privacy when I was teaching.

A financial splurge paid handsome dividends of peace. I bought each of them an inexpensive TV for their bedrooms. Kim had one in the living room which was now her "bedroom." Perhaps parking the kids in front of the TV was frowned upon by family counselors but it was the perfect solution in these circumstances.

Finding something productive for Kim to do all day was another challenge. I bought her a paint-by-number set and she loved it! She painted twenty big pictures over the next few months. I was relieved to see her enjoying something that kept her focused for hours. Unfortunately, painting became impossible when her hands began to shake more from her medications.

The next project I found was a keychain that she could make even with trembling hands. The keychains used cords and beads that were large enough for her to manage. She delighted in going to the craft store and picking out the supplies. She made dozens of these keychains and mounted them on a poster board to sell door to door. I don't know if people actually liked them or bought them out of kindness, but she sold almost all of them! She still remembers taking her $30 from sales to the corner convenience store and blowing the whole wad on junk food!

I could always tell when the voices were very active. She would stop what she was doing and stare into space, listening to something nobody else could hear. Sleep would bring some relief from the tormenting voices, but her dreams were often nightmares. The trauma inflicted by Raul Chapa was relived in her dreams for years after the rapes. The only thing that made either of us feel better was to forgive Raul after every nightmare. This forgiveness took several years to eventually take root in our hearts, but we would say it even if we could not feel it at the moment.

The doctors biggest challenge was finding the best dosage of medication to keep her manageable but still coherent. I remember reading about the side effects of the anti-psychotic medication. The side effects were identical to the symptoms the medication was supposed to help! I asked her psychiatrist about this. Her response was not what I expected. "We are still in the very earliest stages of trying to find the best medications for psychosis. The truth is we have no real way to know if the medication is causing more of the same symptoms. So, we have to adjust dosages to see how the patient responds."

"Oh", I responded. "In other words, they are experiments and guinea pigs?" I still did not fully grasp how little the doctors knew about the effects of these drugs on the brain.

"Pretty much", she admitted. "I may not put it in exactly those terms, but we are doing the best we can." I knew this was true. The doctors were always compassionate and patient as they understood the stress family experiences with this dreadful disease.

The voices were Kim's constant companion and it was impossible to convince her that she didn't have to obey them. I tried reasoning with her. "Honey, I know the voices are very real, but they cannot hurt you. What do you think will happen if you just ignore them and don't obey them?"

"You don't understand Mom. They make me do it." Then she would shut down each conversation with, "I don't want to talk about it anymore." I learned not to push harder when she said that because it seemed to cause her even more inner anguish.

Other than grief, anger was another emotion that surfaced at times which was accompanied by guilt. I knew Kim was very ill and fighting her own battle each day. I admired her courage and faith which kept her motivated to find something to enjoy in her daily life. I was ashamed of myself when I felt angry over something she really could not help. But there were times when I just could not help myself either. My anger flared as she began throwing away all her clothes when the voices commanded it.

"You better not throw away any more of your things," I finally shouted in frustration. "I cannot afford to keep buying you more clothes! If you do it again, I am only buying you one outfit, so you will be naked if you throw that away!"

A few days later a knock at the door startled me when the maintenance man for our apartment complex asked why Kim had wanted to borrow his fishing rod. She had returned it but would not tell him why she needed it. I could not help but laugh when she finally admitted to me what her fishing expedition was all about: "God told me to throw away my makeup, so I threw it in the big dumpster. Then I remembered that I didn't have to live with God, I had to live with Mom, and she was going to be really mad! So, I tried to fish it out of the dumpster."

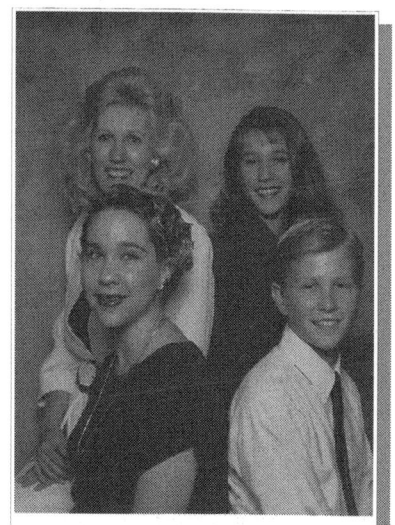

Mom & Rachele in back.
Kim & Keith in front.
Six months before
onset of schizophrenia

She had also started to put on some weight due to the medications which seemed to affect her metabolism. Rachele came crying to me one day after Kim raided her closet looking for something to wear because she had thrown away most of her own clothes. "Mom! She ruined my dress," poor Rachele was crushed. One of her favorite spandex dresses was obviously stretched out of shape when Kim tried to squeeze into it."

"I am so sorry sweetie. I will make sure she doesn't get into your clothes again," I consoled her.

We tried to make the best of it from week to week. I was still grateful she was not wandering the streets of San Antonio like some poor souls who suffer mental illness without a family to protect them.

# Saints walk among us

I sometimes wondered why the voices had only negative things to say. Why couldn't they say, "You're such a great girl." And if they insisted on obedience, how about: "Clean the house for your Mom today." I pity people who lack a well-oiled sense of humor when dealing with mental illness. It was my best therapy.

Some people think I am a very strong person, but Kim is a real super hero when it comes to strength and *uncommon courage*.

In my spiritual quest I discovered there are people who believe in soul groups that live in a higher dimension. They are our soul family. Supposedly, we all decided what our roles would be here on earth. I have fun imagining Kim and I in that scenario:

"OK, which of us is going to be the daughter that goes crazy for most of her life?"

Kim would surely have said, "I'll do it because you are such a sissy when it comes to the really hard stuff."

"Ok, I agree. I get to be the loving mom who everyone thinks is exceptional and strong. Yeah, that is far easier than having to be the crazy one." Maybe I will eventually grow enough spiritually so I can be the crazy one in my next life. I love to laugh at my own jokes.

Thank goodness Tammy Erlanson also had a great sense of humor. Tammy was Kim's case manager, and she became my life line to sanity. She was also responsible for getting Kim on a very new medication that held out real hope for a more manageable life. Tammy has a lifetime of service and was an extraordinary social worker. To really appreciate her you must read a letter of recommendation from one of her former clients (that's what they call patients in the mental health community).

She keeps it to cheer herself up on tough days. It was written when a Bi-Polar patient was experiencing one of his manic phases, and I wholeheartedly agree with his perceptions of Tammy. She thinks the reference to a "local saint" is quite funny, but who says the truth cannot be funny!

I will quote a few paragraphs of his letter.

*"This I write to fully and to the highest possible degree commend and praise the tireless, thorough, and selfless work of Tammy Erlanson. I have been with MHMR, (Mental Health and Mental Retardation) for six years and Ms. Erlanson has been with me the entire span. This is especially outstanding as Tammy earned herself a master degree recently and, praise God!, decided to remain a **local saint**.*

*Tammy's commitment to our community shows that not everyone is only interested in the brass ring or selfish advancement. When I was (chose) to be housebound, Tammy would drive to the house for meetings and she would even stay longer than the allotted time. Tammy is the only reason I became employed while struggling to find the right medication.*

*Ms. Erlanson steps out of her own skin and walks the extra mile, and then another mile. No degree (however high and prestigious) can teach character. I know that Tammy Erlanson would darn near saved this town even with a fourth-grade education. Note that I can be manic and grandiose, but Tammy has always kept me grounded and in touch. I owe MHMR at least one million dollars. I will never be able to pay the debt. But as Tammy shows, heart and soul have no price tag."*

Tammy's note to me regarding that letter is so beautifully expressed, I want to share it.

*"The reason I keep the letter is not only to cheer me up but mostly to remind myself that what I did mattered. It may not matter to the masses, but it mattered to God.*

*Working with the mentally ill did not offer immediate reward because we rarely saw much progress. Our goal was to improve their quality of life and keep them out of the hospital.*

*I think of my time as a case manager like the star fish story.*

**A man walked along the beach throwing star fish back into the ocean, so they would not die. With hundreds of star fish on the beach he was told by friends there were far too many to make a difference. He picked another one up, tossed it in the water and said, "made a difference in that one's life."**

*The clients do not have the ability to thank you because their illness is so incapacitating, and they are just trying to survive. Many families eventually drop out of the picture when they see little or no progress and are overwhelmed by the demands of caring for a chronically-ill loved one.*

*To send a letter like this meant a client took the time to express his gratitude for your hard work and dedication. He really thought about the time and effort I gave him to show that **his life did matter**."*

Tammy is one of many social workers who serve selflessly day in and day out to assist and comfort our mentally ill population. The next time you feel frustrated or angry about the craziness in politics or the world in general, remember Tammy Erlanson and her team of thousands. You will shift immediately from grumpy to grateful.

She reminds us that at the end of our life, the most important thing we can leave behind and what we all desire at the deepest core of our being: *We matter.*

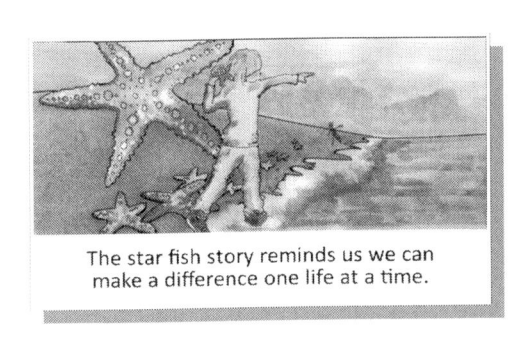

The star fish story reminds us we can make a difference one life at a time.

# The men in my life

As the law suit against the hospital played out with attorneys behind the scenes, I focused on keeping Kim as stable as possible. Finances were always on my mind and Tony Fama from KSAT 12 news had not only helped us with his excellent reporting about the hospital fence, he also connected me with a most unusual man known as "Papa Bear" in San Antonio.

His real name was Robert Edwards and he was the founder of the San Antonio AIDS Foundation. He preferred to be called Papa Bear or just Bear. He looked like a grizzly bear of a man with a long bushy beard that Santa Claus could envy.

Tony said, "I want you to contact Papa Bear. He will help you get the financial aid you need for Kim. He really knows his stuff when it comes to getting deserving people approved for SSI." (Social Security Supplemental Income) I didn't even know this kind of financial aid was available.

It was wonderful to be able to call Papa Bear and tell him Tony Fama had referred us to him. Tony was a well-recognized reporter in our community. Papa Bear didn't hesitate to help, and he handled all the paperwork for us. He had Kim approved in six weeks. This was no small thing because many people pay attorneys to help them get approved and it can take from six months to several years.

He retired in 1991, never having taken a salary for his work. He passed away in 2016. I will honor him in my heart always. After reading Papa Bear's achievements from a San Antonio Aids Foundation website, I thought: "There needs to be more reporting on all the good things people are doing. We are bombarded with so much negative news."

To my delight I have discovered that Tony Fama is doing this! He created 50PLUS PRIME TV NEWS MAGAZINE. He travels the country looking for baby boomers who are making a difference in their communities. He says, "When we find you, and there are millions of you, we like to share your story."

Tony referred me to Papa Bear who made it possible for Kim to get the financial aid which enables her to qualify for medication, doctors care, and housing. I can say *thank you* best by sharing his website address. *50PlusPrime.com* You can also find him on Facebook.

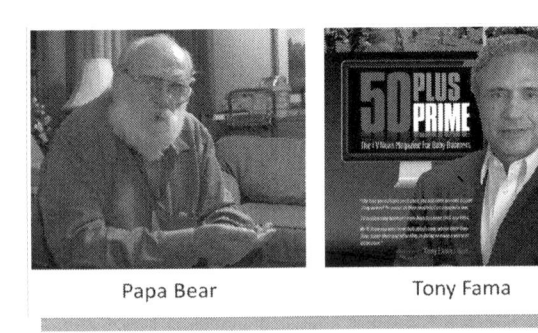

| Papa Bear | Tony Fama |

I would never be where I am today without the help of those two amazing men. Now I was about to meet the man who proved "love at first sight" is not just in fairytales.

I had dated a little and gone to a few clubs for fun, but my heart was at home with my children. "What's out there that is worth forfeiting a good night's sleep Doris?"

"Cheryl, you have to go out with me tonight!" exclaimed Doris, the manager of our apartment complex.

There is a musician I want you to hear. This guy owns a club and he play the guitar, trumpet, keyboard and Sax. He's so cool!"

"Alright! That sounds like a good time! See you tonight!"

The musician was excellent, but he was not the real reason I was there that night.

Rick Wiker asked me to dance and it was the highlight of my entire life when we danced for the first time. I will never forget how he took me in his arms, and I could literally feel the warmth and kindness of his spirit. I don't think I even realized how much my heart needed that affection. I fell in love with him that very first dance. It was much deeper than infatuation or lust. We spoke on the phone daily and our weekends together were the highlight of my week. I was also a little confused because I had been indoctrinated with some traditional Christian teachings that said we should not be "unequally yoked." In Christian communities this meant a "believer" should not marry an "unbeliever."

We should be on the same spiritual wavelength and Rick had no interest in anything spiritual! He wasn't against it, but simply not interested. I reread Corinthians 13, known as the "love chapter" in the Bible. It said, "love is kind, slow to anger, does not envy or boast. It is not arrogant or rude. It doesn't insist on its' own way, etc." Rick embodied all these qualities. I decided this "love" was enough "spirituality" for me. Rick's warmth and affection was like a big glass of refreshing water after a long hike in a very dry desert.

But I was not sure how he would feel about my children, the three most important people in my life. He had been single for many years and had an adult son who lived across the country. There was only one thing I knew for sure. He made me feel loved and I let myself enjoy it without feeling guilty for ignoring the "unequally yoked" advice.

# The eye of the storm

The world within our home often felt like an unpredictable storm. I kept trying to find the eye of the hurricane for some much-needed peace of mind. I could only imagine what it felt like to be in Kim's mind. But I knew more turbulence was in the forecast even during brief moments of calm.

Kim's strong spirit always inspired me because no matter what happened, she seemed able to accept her life as it was and embrace it with her whole heart. She could live moment to moment whereas I seemed to always be searching for something that would improve her future.

Kim's case manager, Tammy, had been researching a new drug called Clozaril. It had some risky, life-threatening side effects. But it also had the potential to greatly help schizophrenics. With Tammy's encouragement, Kim began this life changing medication. The pharmaceutical company provided the medication free of charge for patients who could not afford it.

I began to reflect on the timing of past events and realized there was a huge silver lining in the hospital's decision not to repair the fence at that time. If the hospital had fixed the fence immediately, I would never have filed the law suit which became the catalyst for getting Kim out of the hospital. She would have lived the rest of her life in the State hospital's long-term care unit. She would never get to try this new medication. It was not available to hospital patients because it was extremely expensive.

I was willing to accept this new drug's health risks because the anti-psychotic meds she was currently on could cause permanent damage to the nervous system, resulting in constant twitching. Kim responded beautifully to the medication and became much easier to manage. The only anxiety I felt concerned the required weekly blood test designed to reveal a lowered white blood cell count. If this happened, the medication would be discontinued because the patient could die from a severely compromised immune system. This was so discouraging for those who had improved significantly while on the medication. Removing it was a return to mental mayhem and madness.

I began to relax a bit when Kim's blood tests were stable. The tests were done weekly for years and thereafter, every two weeks. Today it is a monthly test. These are powerful, brain altering drugs. Mental health professionals diligently monitor symptoms and side effects.

Tammy explains the situation which allowed Kim to benefit from this medication:

*"The typical antipsychotic medications had been on the market for years. While many of them were somewhat successful, they also successfully sucked the life out of patients. The side effects were almost as debilitating as the disease. In the 90's we heard about a new antipsychotic medication called Clozaril that was successfully treating patients with schizophrenia. However, it was so expensive that patients could not afford it or the required weekly blood test. The test was mandatory because the medication could lower the white*

*blood cells. This side effect would make the patient vulnerable to infections which could lead to death due to a compromised immune system.*

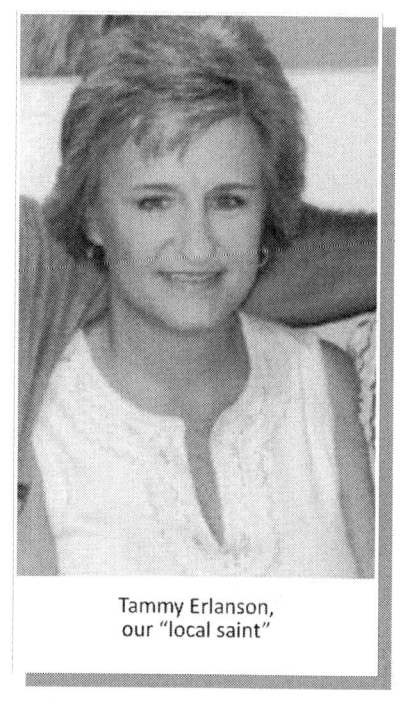

Tammy Erlanson,
our "local saint"

*While MHMR[1] centers provided medications, they could not afford this new medication. All pharmaceutical companies have patient assistance programs to help the indigent population who could not otherwise afford their medication.*

*Kim was one of three patients who found relief from this medication after I applied for approval on her behalf. It was truly life changing for all three of them. The illness was not*

1 Acronym for Mental Health and Mental Retardation. This was later changed to Mental Health and Developmentally Disabled, MHDD.

*cured but it helped tremendously to calm the terrible battle going on in their heads. While maintenance of the medication was significant, the benefits were even greater.*

I am forever grateful for Tammy's help which allowed us some relief from the storm which had often threatened to overwhelm us.

# I totally lose it

When Kim came home from the hospital, I could no longer supplement our income with work outside the home, so I took on a huge teaching load. I also had a new man in my life that made those endorphins fire all day long. I was so happy!

Just when I thought life was turning around with a wonderful man in my life and Kim's improvement, a new crisis was brewing. I should have been aware of the undercurrents of anxiety and frustration Keith was suffering, but he had never given me any problems. For some reason Keith began to turn into a back talking and belligerent teenager. He spent more and more time in his room and there was a growing venom in his remarks. I had never experienced this hostility from him. In retrospect, his anger, anxiety and frustration are completely understandable. He did not have a father he could relate to since their temperaments were total opposites. He needed a home that felt calm with a sense of security and normal routine. Instead, he could only find much needed peace behind the locked bedroom door, which was sometimes banged on by his crazy sister.

But I didn't have time to analyze the situation with so many other irons in the fire.

Toby and I were preparing for her annual dance recital. Some of my students would play the piano for her dancers. This was a challenging performance for my students because they had to be perfect with their rhythms and tempos. Dancers depended on this precision and accuracy.

As the dance recital drew near, I found out Rachele's high school graduation was scheduled for the same time as the dance recital! I panicked and felt very anxious because I could not abandon my students during the recital. How could I tell Rachele I would miss her graduation? I had missed all her band performances because I was teaching. I tried to make it up to her by planning a small party after the graduation ceremony. She never complained but I knew my absence would hurt and I had no band aid big enough for her hurting heart.

Life had become a series of problems to solve. It was much easier when I accepted that fact and used my energy to solve the problem instead of stewing about it. That day, my biggest dilemma was what to do with Kim during the graduation. She really wanted to go, so I told Keith he needed to sit with her and keep an eye on her.

This was way more than a self-conscious fifteen-year-old boy could handle. He was mortified and refused to help. His sister would draw attention to him as she constantly shook her feet and could not sit still for long. It was obvious to anyone that she was not normal, and just the thought of taking her to the graduation made him cringe with embarrassment.

I couldn't ask Rick to help since Kim would feel uncomfortable with someone she didn't know well. He was still living in San Antonio and we only saw each other on the weekends. Kim ended up staying at home during the graduation. She didn't complain but she still remembers how much she wanted to go.

One of the most valuable things I have learned through observing Kim's life is to gracefully accept life's imperfections, disappointments and challenges. She has an unusual ability to simply let life be whatever it is at the moment, without resistance. I didn't have this ability at the time. I would give anything to be able to turn back the clock and rewrite this chapter. I totally lost it that day! Poor Keith became the victim of my emotional meltdown.

"This is the last straw Keith. You think you have it tough here? You need to find out how good you have it here." My frustration turned to anger as I vented on him. I packed up his clothes and sent him to live with his father, knowing full well the emotional boot camp would either make or break him.

There were probably books available about how to deal with rebellious teens, but I doubted there were any that addressed rebellious teens with a crazy and bossy older sister. I didn't have a clue how to handle this situation and used humor to offset the shock waves. "If you kids give me any more grief, I am going to dig a puberty pit and put you in it. I'll throw bananas down occasionally and let you out when you turn eighteen and are fit for society again!" For some reason I was the only one who thought that was hilarious.

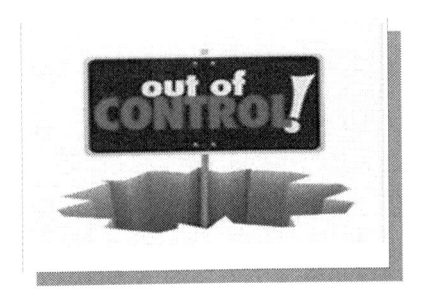

By this time, I would do just about anything to have peace at home. Emotionally detached, I heartlessly sent my tender-hearted son away. What kind of mother does that? Survival mode was my state of mind and I lived in it for several years.

Kim now had Keith's room and she was glad to have a bed to replace the couch she had slept on for months. I went to bed thinking, "problem solved." I was becoming a highly efficient problem-solving machine.... oops I meant mother.

The only predictable thing about schizophrenia is its unpredictability. We never knew what might cause Kim to become highly agitated. Perhaps it was adjusting medication levels, hormones or both. Kim went into a rage one day out of the blue. I have no memory of what the issue was, but she was up in my face screaming, "I can't hear you, blah, blah, blah!!" She held her ears, screamed in my face and shoved me hard which was really unnerving.

I could not reason with her and calm her down. The situation was escalating, and I had to do something fast because my piano students were due to arrive shortly! I hesitated to call their parents because I did not want to tell them I had a paranoid schizophrenic daughter at home. This was a small town and I would lose students and our livelihood if parents felt their children were trying to learn in an unstable home environment.

I called Kim's case manager, Tammy, and begged her to come get Kim after explaining the need for immediate help in this emergency. I was not prepared for what came next. "Cheryl, you are going to have to put all of her belongings outside, so she is legally homeless. We are not allowed to give assistance and get her the medical care she needs unless she is homeless."

"Oh, dear God in heaven! How am I going to do this? Why, why, why?" I didn't have time to process it with my students due on the doorstep within the hour. I quickly packed her clothes and toiletries in several large trash bags because I didn't even have suit cases. I put my daughter outside the door with the trash bags and locked it behind me.

I thought Tammy was on the way to pick her up, but Kim ran next door and used the neighbor's phone to call a pastor in town. He picked her up and eventually she was sent to live with her father. I felt sorry for him. He had never lived with her since she became ill after the divorce. But it was also a relief to know he had put her ahead of his ministry, which had always been his first priority.

I had no parents to call for emotional support. My mom had passed away and dad was now married to a woman that had no interest in a relationship with his children.

The day I put Kim and her few belongings outside was a deeply depressing low point in my life. It was a pain so deep that even friends could not comfort me. Love could not comfort me, and hope washed away with my tears of grief. I clung desperately to faith that life could not feel this bad forever. I cried myself to sleep that night with prayers for God's grace to get us through another day.

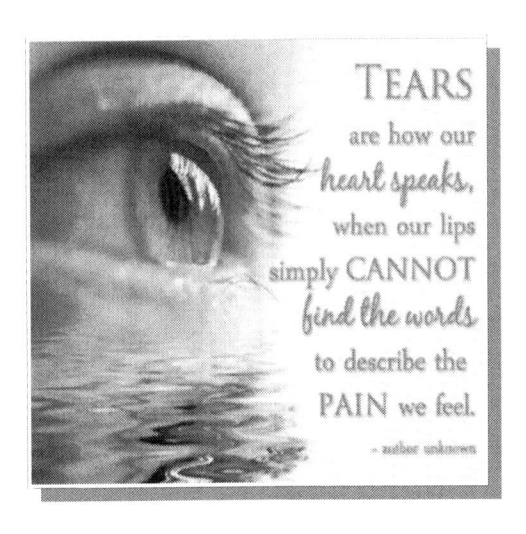

TEARS
are how our
*heart speaks,*
when our lips
simply CANNOT
*find the words*
to describe the
PAIN we feel.

– author unknown

# The good, the bad, and the ugly

Rick and I met in April and we were having a wonderful time dating on the weekends. Keith and Kim were now living with their Dad. Rachele went off to college that Fall, creating a space without any children at home. Rick moved in with me and it felt like a real honeymoon away from an overwhelming life.

There was one thing that started to bother me. Rick was a heavy drinker. But he never seemed unsteady and didn't slur his words. He seemed to come to life when he had a few drinks and we had so much fun that I didn't see it as a big problem.

However, dating and living together were two very different things. I loved how easy he was to live with, but I could not keep up with him on the weekends. One Saturday night I remember wanting to go to bed. It was almost two in the morning and Rick wanted to dance me around the bedroom! I wanted to settle down into a more normal lifestyle, so I asked him to please cut back his drinking.

He patiently explained one more time, something I had refused to grasp: "I tried to tell you I should not drink at all because I am an alcoholic. I can't seem to quit once I start." I was so naïve. I had no experience with alcoholism. I had observed my parents having a martini when my Dad came home from work. And I might indulge in two glasses of wine. Maybe he just needed to learn how to say," two drinks and no more."

We were married in November and when our schedules allowed, we went to Cancun, Mexico with an all-inclusive vacation deal. The package price included all the food and drinks you could consume. One evening I went to bed early not feeling well. I asked him to please not drink too much when he left the room. I woke up at three am and went to look for him. I found him having a wonderful time with his new buddies. He was delighted to see me.

"Hi honey! Come meet Bob, and Mike and the guys! Guys, meet my beautiful girl!"

They were having a jolly old time, but I was livid. He had promised he would not drink too much and come to bed a little earlier that night. I took his drink and threw it in his face. I was furious! However, he was not angry. He followed me back to the room like a shamed puppy.

The following afternoon we sat on the bed and cried. I wondered how all this could turn out so bad when he was such a good person. The ugly truth: he was an alcoholic. I was in love with an alcoholic and I was in a state of shock. How could I be so naïve?

I thought of my children. They were always my first priority. How could I tell them I had married an alcoholic? They would lose all respect for me. I would lose all respect for myself. I wept as I quietly but resolutely told him I had to file for divorce when we got home. I simply could not do this to the kids. They would never in a million years understand their Mom marrying an alcoholic.

He cried too and simply said, "Then I quit." He never took a drink again and we have been married for twenty-five years!

I have enjoyed imagining an unseen world of the spirit where this unlikely partnership might have been created. There were two angels who worked in the match making department. One thought it was a good match but the other one wasn't so sure.

"No, no, no. You cannot put these two together! She knows nothing about alcohol, and he knows nothing about church. What are you thinking!"

"They are perfect for each other. He loves her enough to give up drinking and she needs his warm heart."

"Can't you find another guy with a warm heart who is a better match for her?"

"It isn't that easy to find one with a warm heart big enough for *her and her three children*. Trust me, this is a very good match."

There is a verse in the bible that says, "For where your treasure is, there your heart will be also." Rick's love and support has been demonstrated constantly through his financial generosity to our children. They are not just my children anymore. I hate to think what our life would be without him.

What if I hadn't given him a second chance when he said: "Then I quit." What if I had researched alcoholics and their relapses? I was naïve enough to take him at his word. *It turned out to be one of the best decisions of my life.* Never underestimate the power of love. It can enable us to overcome almost any challenge if we don't become "enablers" of self-destructive behavior. It's crucial to be able to discern the difference.

Kim left her dad's home shortly after moving there. She now qualified for a HUD subsidized apartment. Rick furnished her entire apartment and she loved having her own place. And I have discovered more about selfless unconditional love through our marriage than I ever did in a church pew.

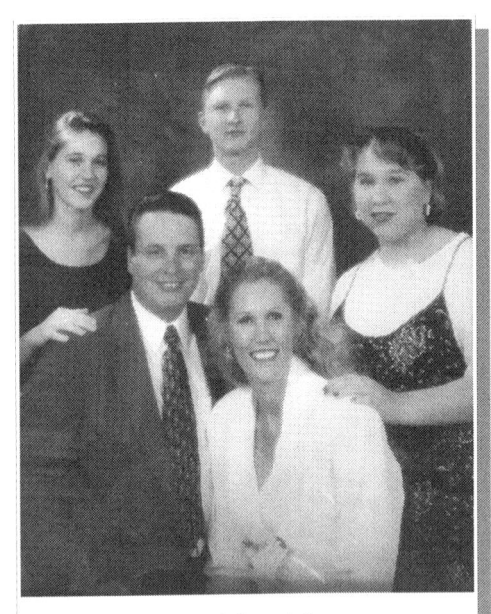

From left to right,
Rachele, Keith, Kim
Rick and Cheryl

# Michigan miracle

Keith traveled with his dad that summer and I hoped they were getting along. Rachele called me one day and said, "Mom, please let Keith come home. He is miserable and struggling with depression. I am really worried about him. He feels hopeless and trapped and is going to try and find a gun so he can end it all."

I was devastated and realized the emotional boot camp that I predicted would make or break him was breaking him. I struggled to forgive myself for putting him though this. I asked him to come home and he gratefully returned. He was once again back to his old self that never gave me any problems and I loved having him home.

We didn't know it at the time but travel and a whole new life was on the horizon! This life would include a wonderful new apartment, with a bus line for greater independence, a top-notch mental health support team, new friends, and a real sense of community for Kim.

Rick was a computer programmer, working in the corporate office of Builders Square, under the larger K-Mart corporate structure. His excellent skill set did not go unnoticed by one of its Vice Presidents, who moved to Ann Arbor, Michigan to expand the Information Technology department for Borders Books. He offered Rick an exciting employment opportunity which took advantage of Rick's programming skills and valued business analysis.

I discovered Michigan had some wonderful benefits for Kim that were unavailable in Texas. Borders paid for our move to Michigan and covered the cost of breaking Kim's lease, allowing her to move with us.

Keith was fine with the idea and Rachele stayed in her dorm at St Mary's University in San Antonio. She was dating a young man who shared her enjoyment of music. It tugged at my heart strings to leave her, but I knew this move was a wonderful opportunity to give Kim a better life and we were excited for Rick too. I had no idea that the December move was also going to manifest a Christmas miracle that has brought me much comfort and joy for many years.

I enjoyed imagining what my ideal life would look like if I could create it out of thin air or use a magic wand to materialize my dream home. It would be a cabin in the woods with large windows and a cozy fireplace. But that was a pipe dream since I could not live in the country and teach piano. Students needed a more centrally located teacher.

We looked at apartments for rent when we arrived in Ann Arbor, but they all felt sterile and we would be cramped for space. I decided to look for a house to rent. My heart raced with excitement when I looked at the very first home on my list. It sat on a hill with rustic railroad tie stairs surrounded by woods. It had floor to ceiling wall to wall windows with a deck overlooking the surrounding property. It had a cozy stone fireplace!

And most miraculous of all, it was located right between Ypsilanti and Ann Arbor, near a main thoroughfare that made it an ideal location for piano students from both cities! The owners lived behind the house and had purchased it as a rental property. They were a lovely senior couple, who wanted to rent to us as much as we were eager to live in this dream house. The moving company had our furniture delivered within one week and we enjoyed a snowy winter, warmed by the wood burning fireplace.

Several years later they surprised us with a proposal. "Every renter has wanted to buy the house from us. But we decided we would like to have you as our lifetime neighbors and want to know if you would like to buy it?"

"Oh gosh yes! But we don't have enough money for a down payment," we sadly responded.

"That is fine. We can offer it as a land contract, and you can pay us what you can afford."

So, for a very minimal down payment and affordable monthly mortgage, we were ecstatic, first-time home owners. This home continues to warm our hearts and the fireplace has been enjoyed by many friends and family. Tom Crosley, the attorney for the law suit, remembers sitting by the cozy fire when he flew up for Kim's taped deposition.

That law suit was still in the background of our lives, but life moves on despite the ever so slow wheels of justice.

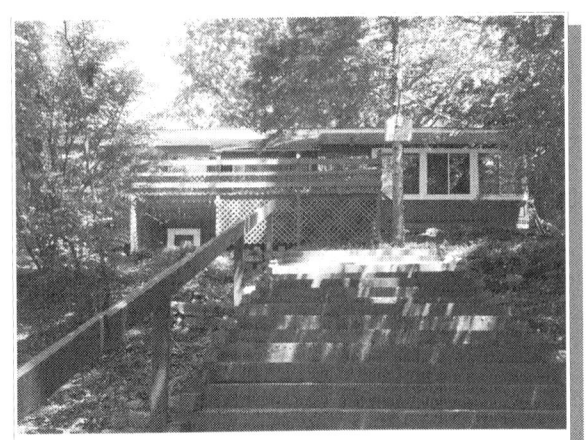

Our cabin in the woods in the middle of town!

# We won the battle but lost the war

Shortly after our move to Michigan, the court case began to move forward after seeming stagnant for the previous year. I am not sure what lawyers accomplished during that time, but they managed to generate huge boxes of paperwork in files that they eventually delivered to the courtroom on dollies!

Our attorney, Tom Crosley, was very protective of Kim and made sure she was not put into a stressful situation. Courtroom testimony would put her at risk of destabilizing. He arranged to have her deposition videotaped in our living room. A court recorder and attorney for the state of Texas flew to Michigan to ask the questions needed for their defense. Tom also flew up, at his own expense!

The thing I remember most vividly was how the State of Texas attorney worded questions in such a way Kim's responses could be used against her. For example, "Isn't it true that you went willingly with Mr. Chapa when you left the hospital grounds and you willingly had sexual relations with him?"

Kim has a very innocent spirit which shone brightly in the deposition when they tried to paint a much darker picture of her. "I liked being married. He gave me a ring and said we were married. But I didn't want to have *sex* with him!"

At one point I felt the court recorder's embarrassment as she felt bad for Kim who was obviously a very naïve, mentally disabled young woman who had been violated. This felt like another violation of her innocent spirit, but Kim answered every question with the truth as she remembered it. I have always been proud of her integrity.

Jury selection was another interesting experience. Prospective jurors were asked questions by both attorneys. The State attorney asked, "Have any of you had previous experience or knowledge of someone who was a patient at the State Hospital and was off the hospital grounds without permission?" I was shocked and surprised at how many raised their hands! They were immediately dismissed.

The trial took place from December 10th through the 16th of 1996. The State's defense is explained in Tom Crosley's summary of the trial.

*"The State hospital claimed that the fence was not for security, and therefore, a hole in the fence did not pose an unreasonable risk of harm to the plaintiff. The defendant also contended that the hole in the fence could not have proximately caused the plaintiff's injuries."*

It did not sit well with the jury when they were told the fence was not there for security. These were court committed patients which meant they were considered a threat to themselves or others. I imagine they were as incredulous as I was to see the hospital claim the fence was not for security.

With Tom's excellent presentation of our case, and a jury that had common sense, we won the trial. The jury found the defendant 100% negligent and awarded actual damages of approximately $97,000. Of course, the State appealed this decision and the jury verdict was reversed on the issue of proximate cause. I will let Tom explain exactly what this is in layman's terms.

*"I always felt like the courts changed the rules in the middle of the game. While our case was in queue for the appeals court, the Texas Supreme Court ruled on another case that would make our case a lost cause. A man had escaped a psychiatric ward through a door that had been left unlocked. He ran into the street and was killed. The court determined that the* **State could only be sued if the property itself was the direct cause of the injury**.

*For example, if he had run down some stairs and the stairs collapsed due to disrepair then the State would be liable. An unlocked door could be negligence but the door itself did not injure the man.*

*The State has immunity regarding negligence even if it is obvious to all concerned. They ruled that the fence itself did not damage Kim, so the jury verdict was overturned."*

I believe the immunity the government gives itself is unjust. If a private hospital had been responsible, they would have been accountable for obvious negligence. I may have lost faith in our justice system, but my faith in the decency of individuals has been strengthened. There is so much good within people. Tom called me several years after the final verdict. "I just want you to know that I drive the perimeter of the hospital compound occasionally and *they are keeping that fence repaired!"*

He said he wished they could have done more, but thanks to Tom, *I believe we accomplished what we set out to do.* Tom spent a huge amount of his time, energy and money without any financial compensation. He did this because he is a man of integrity with a sincere desire to serve his community. **His** *work made a difference to the hospital because they keep the fence repaired now.*

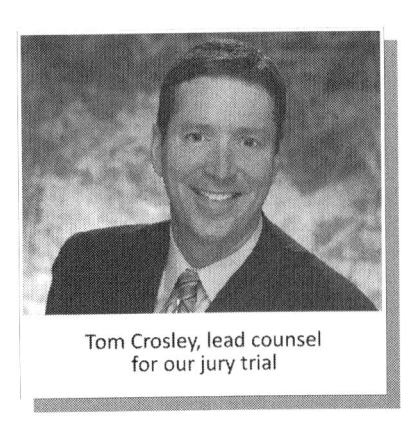

Tom Crosley, lead counsel
for our jury trial

# Faith, hope & love

There are three eternal elements, *faith, hope and love*. Our lives literally embody these spiritual truths. We can be *strengthened* by them or *diminished* if we forget to rely on them. They are magnified when families cope with a chronic non-curable illness. We demonstrate *faith* by knowing we can handle whatever each day brings to us. When it is a crazy day, we *hope* tomorrow will be better. We *love* our mentally ill children so much that we are willing to do whatever it takes to make their life a little easier.

Moving to another state is exciting but also a huge upheaval in routines as you leave behind everyone and everything that is familiar. It is even more challenging when a mentally ill family member is part of the move. This is when having helpful case managers and doctors is not just comforting but essential. Records must be sent to the new support team and medications secured. This was especially important with the weekly blood test that was required for patients on Clozaril.

I often put great *faith* in the social workers who made our world manageable. Their genuine *love* for the mentally ill always gave me *hope* for a better future for Kim. This *faith, hope and love* was rewarded when we had to leave our wonderful Case Manager, Tammy in Texas.

Kim enjoyed the move to Michigan, and I was so grateful for Rick's patience and generous support. She wore headphones to listen to music because it seemed to help drown out the voices that were her constant companion. The Clozaril helped calm her, but the voices were never completely silent.

We settled into a routine that included the weekly blood test and attending a support facility called Full Circle Community. They met in an old church and provided socialization, meals and group therapy. This was a safe place for people with mental health conditions to share their lives and challenges with others without any embarrassment. Kim has belonged to the Full Circle community for twenty years. Recently the community asked her to be their Board Secretary. She was elected and is proud to be serving in this capacity.

When you cannot work or drive, finding such a purpose is incredibly fulfilling. She was so happy when she called me one day, "Mom! They voted me onto the Board at Full Circle!" I was thrilled to hear the excitement in her voice. "I feel like I really have a place in life here. I feel like I really belong."

I realized how much she held inside because she had never told me that she had felt this need to belong somewhere. The severely mentally ill may have scrambled brains but their spirit is very much intact. So, it makes sense that they want to be useful and part of a community just like you and me.

She was always excited to try anything new that would challenge her and provide a sense of belonging. She worked as a volunteer at a local thrift shop and I enrolled her for some easy piano and dance classes at a community college. She enjoyed them tremendously so it was time to see how much she could handle with more challenging classes. An entry level computer class started out well but as soon as she had to work on her own, the stress began to affect her. I think I was always more disappointed than she was when she suffered a setback.

Our community provided a psychiatric annual evaluation which was a three-hour test administered by a psychiatrist. Kim had the same results for three years. She was able to handle intellectual concepts, but any stress would destabilize her which could lead to a psychotic break. The results were sad, but very helpful for me. I learned not to push her too hard.

Kim befriended Monica at Full Circle because she noticed Monica had a Jesus pin on her blouse. When Monica moved into her own apartment, she invited Kim to see it. The idea of living independently took root and Kim talked us into applying for an apartment of her own.

Chidester Place Apartments are HUD subsidized and thanks to Tony Fama and Papa Bear, Kim was an SSI recipient and qualified to live in the facility. This was an exciting new adventure! Rick once again paid to have her apartment furnished with a new bed, living room furniture, wall hangings, dishes, new everything!

I remember the night we left her there for her first night in her own place. She was excited, but I was apprehensive about how she would do on her own. I quit worrying after I called the next morning to see how she slept.

"I slept like I was in heaven! I love my new apartment!"

Here are the three eternal elements again. I now trusted (*faith*) that she would do fine, *hoped* it would last and *loved* seeing her so happy!

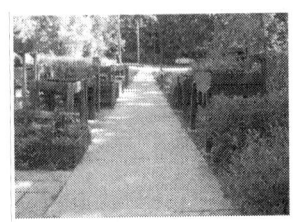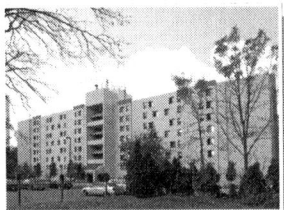

Chidester Place provides apartments for the disabled in Ypsilanti, Michigan. Residents enjoy creating a garden for fresh vegetables!

# True hope

Each week I took Kim grocery shopping. These trips usually brought up another emotion that disturbed me. I thought I should be more mature and was secretly ashamed of myself for feeling embarrassed by Kim's behavior when we shopped together. If I was in another aisle picking up something on her list, I would hear her yelling loudly from another aisle!

"Mom, do we have enough money to get these cookies?" Or, "Where are you Mom? I need help finding the ketchup."

She had no self-awareness of how inappropriate the yelling was and when I explained it, she would promise not to do it again. That promise was always forgotten by the next shopping trip. I decided to always stay next to her to avoid the embarrassment.

When driving, I gripped the steering wheel firmly because I feared the voices might tell her to grab the wheel and cause an accident. I developed an ability to analyze worst case scenarios in my mind so I would have a plan in place if needed.

I also made sure her medication containers were filled correctly. She was handling life on her own reasonably well, but the voices were now making her life miserable. She always enjoyed reading but the voices now put a stop to this. They also made her stand up and sit back down constantly. It made it impossible for her to enjoy watching a show on

TV. Telling her to ignore the voices made no impact at all.

When medication adjustments did not help, I began to look for something in the alternative medical field or through nutrition. A friend told me about a company that was having tremendous success with a nutritional supplement called *True Hope*.

The founder of this company, Anthony Stephan, lost his wife when she committed suicide after years of struggling with severe depression. Several of his children were also diagnosed as Bi- Polar. He developed a combination of nutrients which has improved the life of thousands of people suffering from mental illness. You can hear the story of his family and his discovery of this nutritional support on the video at his website, ***truehope.com***

I decided to call this company and after consulting with its counselors I realized the name of this company was perfect. For the first time in our struggle with schizophrenia I had true hope. I brought Kim home to begin a slow process of weaning her off the medications and replacing them with the supplements recommended by the counselors.

We diligently completed the daily charts provided by the company, monitoring every symptom. This allowed a computer graph to be created which showed exactly when it was time to cut back the medication ever so slightly. Pill cutters were used to shave off 1/8th of a pill.

The counselors explained what was going to happen next and I was always amazed at how accurate they were. Many of these phone counselors had been diagnosed with severe depression or bi-polar and were now living life completely free of the symptoms that had created such devastation in their lives.

We watched Kim's improvement from month to month with joy and amazement. The voices greatly diminished. She seemed to be much more present in conversations, probably because she no longer had the competing background noise in her head.

One very significant day, she played a card game that had been impossible for her just six months prior to beginning the True Hope program. I was elated and shared the progress with her doctor, who seemed happy but also talked about how powerful the placebo effect could be. This continues to be a source of frustration for me. Getting medical doctors and alternative nutritional practitioners to work together seems as hopeless as getting the politicians from both sides of the isle to work together.

After nine months of the True Hope regimen, Kim was almost completely off medication and doing well enough that I thought she could return to her apartment. She was also excited to gain back her independence.

If I had known what was about to happen, I would have never let her go.

> *H. O. P. E.*
> *Hold*
> *On*
> *Pain*
> *Ends*

# Hope deferred makes the heart sick

Kim and I continued to do the daily charting for the True Hope program, only we did it over the phone now. Symptoms were rated by numbers one through ten. Lower numbers indicated a lessening of the symptoms. I thought things were going well until we received a call at two am one cold winter night.

"Mrs. Wiker? Is this Kim Koehler's Mother?" the police officer asked with urgency.

"Yes! What is going on? Is she OK?"

Waking up to a call like that makes your imagination run wild. Kim's friend, Monica, had recently died because she wandered outside on a freezing night. They found her body the next day. I was grateful Kim was alive because she was found so far away from her apartment.

"We found her wandering by the side of the interstate in Romulus."

"Romulus!", I was panicking. "How did she get there? That is at least ten miles from where she lives!"

"She says she walked but she is pretty incoherent, and we need you to come pick her up."

We were heartbroken on that trip to the police station. Something had gone drastically wrong. Kim seemed to be growing strong and stable. This felt like a devastating earthquake, collapsing everything she had accomplished in the last year.

She went with us willingly, but we could not communicate with her. She babbled crazy, confused thoughts and we took her directly to the hospital. Her treatment was now completely out of my hands and the doctors put her back on the medications that had taken me almost a year to wean her off. I knew I didn't have the strength left to try the nutrients again and feared I could get into legal trouble if her doctors felt I was endangering her by removing the prescribed medication.

After she became reasonably stable, I found out what had happened. She had developed diarrhea which I was unaware of at the time. If the True Hope counselors had known, they would have been able to help. But Kim was the only one who knew, and she never mentioned it. She didn't realize how the diarrhea would affect her body's absorption of the supplements.

How did I miss the signs that she was decompensating? I was feeling unusually fatigued and sometimes waited in the car as she shopped for her groceries. She held it together for the few minutes we were together, hiding her descent into madness. She also informed me that when we were charting over the phone, she did not tell me when her symptoms began to get worse.

"Mom, I didn't want to disappoint you. You were so happy that I was getting better, so I didn't want to make you sad."

"It's okay sweetie. Tomorrow will be a better day."

Proverbs 13:12 says: "hope deferred makes the heart sick." I was heart sick, just as proverbs predicted. But *faith* that tomorrow will bring another reason to *love* and laugh makes me *hope* again and again and again.

# Life returns to normal

Stabilizing after a psychotic break takes time and I was grateful when life returned to normal. Kim was now back on the standard drug regimen and it took months to get the medications in balance, given her unique brain situation. One day I went to her apartment and found her toiletries in the refrigerator, bread and other kitchen items were in the linen closet and under the bathroom sink. Toothpaste was under the bed. This chaos must have seemed logical to her confused brain.

I began to realize how much courage it required to face each day with so much mental chaos. We associate courage with policemen, fire fighters, and our military men in battle. But Kim continually amazed me with her **uncommon courage**, fighting for some semblance of a normal life, when her brain was often sabotaging every effort.

At one-point she felt a need to change something in her environment and wanted to check out the group homes as a possible option. It didn't take her long to realize how fortunate she was to have such a spacious apartment. The group homes were depressing. We looked at a tiny bedroom with a closet half the size of the one in her apartment. A small shabby dresser occupied the room. The stained mattress filled the room with an offensive, foul odor of urine. The living room area was cramped, and the residents stared vacantly at the

TV. The people who managed the home had a much nicer living area, off limits to the residents.

She felt deep gratitude again for her apartment. However, it had also become a scary place in one regard. We had to remove the pictures from the walls because they were talking to her and threatening her. I can only imagine how terrifying it would be to get up each day to walls that seemed to come alive with threatening commands. She would slap herself in the face as commanded and hit her head against the wall. I felt helpless but even worse, she felt helpless to resist the commands and robotically obeyed.

It finally dawned on me that we could give Kim the change she needed and resolve the picture problem at the same time. Her sister, Rachele, made a trip from her home in Ohio to do a complete apartment makeover. She found an excellent entertainment center in a garage sale and installed it, along with lamps and other furnishings she collected for the makeover. Rachele's best idea was to create beautiful walls requiring no pictures of any kind. She used large fabric panels framed with molding to line the walls, creating very elegant walls!

Rick generously provided new living room furniture, TV and DVD player. Kim stayed with Rick and me, as Rachele worked day and night to create a dream apartment. Kim's delight with the big reveal made it all worthwhile.

"OH MY! This is like a gorgeous hotel!" she squealed with pure joy. This change was just what she needed, and she loved keeping her new home in good order. I asked Kim the other day if she ever wished she had a roommate. She replied emphatically: "No way! I get up when I want, watch TV when I want, eat when I want. I don't have to wait to use the bathroom and can go downstairs to talk to people when I want to."

Kim feels deep gratitude for the simple things most of us take for granted. I realized she was happier than many people I knew who had no brain issues at all!

Kim's HUD subsidized apartment with fabric wall panels!

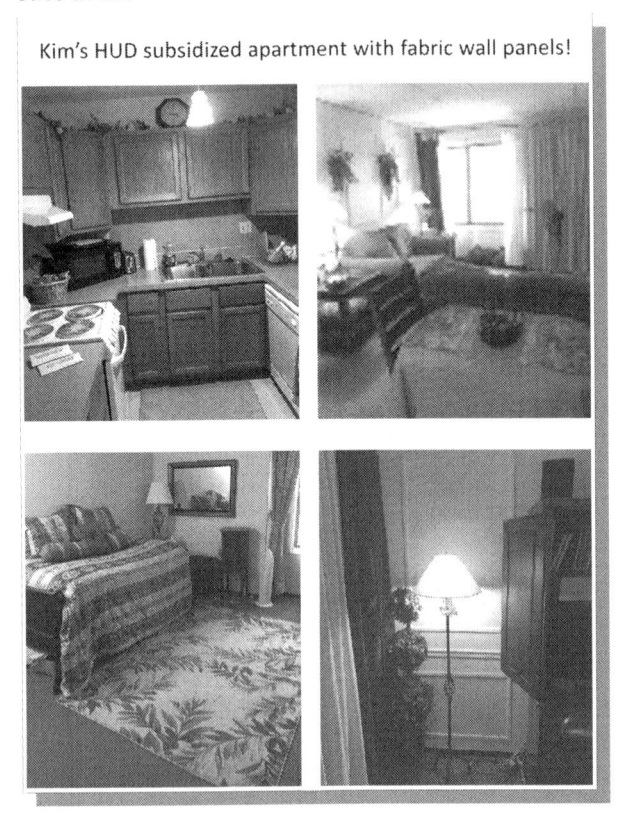

# Caregiver crisis!

Just when life seemed to be on the upswing, my health took a nose dive.

"Rick! Come help me!" I was shaking with shock and fear. We were eating dinner and suddenly nausea overwhelmed me. Running to the bathroom, I was horrified to see the bowl fill with bright red blood. I felt dizzy and woozy on the way to the emergency room. Fortunately, we were only five minutes from the nearest hospital where I was given a blood transfusion.

Years ago, I had contracted hepatitis C from a hospital in Mexico. All three of my children were born in Mexico during twelve years of missionary service. The genotype I contracted was very resistant to the available treatment, so I ate a healthy diet and hoped for the best. I had no symptoms until this terrifying experience.

The hepatitis virus attacked my spleen causing it to grow new veins which were attaching to the stomach. One of the fragile veins had burst, causing life-threatening bleeding. My liver also suffered from cirrhosis which I did not realize at that time. I always assumed any fatigue was related to the stress of caring for a chronically ill daughter.

Due to complications from two surgeries, it took several years to get back on my feet. Rick literally embodied divine unconditional love throughout the entire ordeal. When an infection set in after surgery, I was sent to a rehabilitation facility for several months. No matter how tired he was after a long day at work, he would show up to massage my feet. When he was not there, he was at home doing laundry to bring me fresh pajamas. He bought me a new pair for every day of the week! When I was finally well enough to come home, he served meals to me in the special recliner he bought. It raised me up so I could stand without help and make it to the bathroom. He made sure I knew how much he loved me. Love like that is so healing on many levels. I was finally free of this life-threatening virus in 2015 through a new drug developed for the genotype I had.

*During this time a whole new level of support was also available for Kim.*

What happens to a mentally ill person when their caregiver is disabled? If you are fortunate enough to live in my Michigan town, the community mental health support team sends in Saints, disguised as social workers. Kim struggled to take her medication as prescribed at times, so a social worker arrived at her apartment *every day* to be sure she was taking the medications correctly. Since I could no longer take her grocery shopping or to doctor appointments, the state supplied an aide who took my place, for very little financial reward.

As Kim ages, her mind tends to get confused more often, and this aide now helps with laundry, cooking or cleaning when needed. I honestly don't know how we would manage without this support. Hopefully, this book will bring greater awareness concerning needs of our citizens with a mental health condition. Too often, governments cut their budgets for the mentally ill support. This should **never** happen. *This is something politicians on both sides of the aisle can agree upon.*

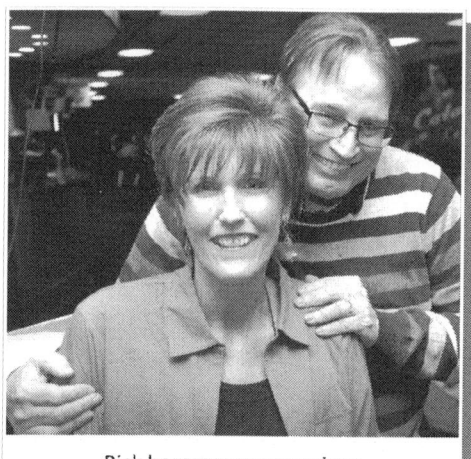

Rick becomes my caregiver.

# Outpatient care – a national disgrace

The evolution of mental health care has been erratic at best. At one point it was decided patients would fare better in a warm family environment, rather than a cold institution.

Deinstitutionalization started in the 1950's and continued for decades. The goal was to improve patient care, but the result was actually the opposite. Families were often not prepared to handle the needs of the mentally ill, and many didn't have access to resources or support from the professional psychiatric community.

Some patients did not have supportive homes to return to. As a result, those whose families could not care for them, and who could not afford private mental health care, often faced abuse at home, became homeless, or were incarcerated.

The number of people in state-funded mental institutions was down from 560,000 in the 1950s, to 130,000 in the 1980s. The number continued to drop as institutions lost funding, and insurance companies cut back their coverage for in-patient mental health care. [2]

Kim is one of the most fortunate patients, surrounded by a supportive family and our community

---

2    Excerpt from Mental Health Care: Past and Present (worldoffemale.com)

mental health care team. As a recipient of monthly SSI, (supplemental security income) she qualifies for Medicaid which covers all her medical care and enables her to live in HUD subsidized housing.

The Full Circle Community Center moved from the church to a wonderful new facility, providing invaluable assistance. They serve lunch to 25 or 30 people every day. Their food budget is supplemented through Food Gatherers who provide low cost or no cost food items for breakfast, lunch and snacks.

Members can relax in a lovely TV room or read magazines and books. They can play pool and games in other activity rooms. There are arts and crafts available and bingo. They give Kim and others a place to socialize and receive compassion and encouragement. Once a month they have Birthday Cake Friday, celebrating everyone's birthday for the month. Some of the members do not have families to celebrate with so the Full Circle community has become their "family."

There are three full time employees and two part time employees. Faith Nichols is the Director who works closely with her Assistant Director, Cheryl Weber. Joe Manney drives and maintains the van and offers support wherever needed. Roz and Elizabeth are part time employees. *As wonderful as this sounds, I was disheartened to discover they have had no increase in funding for fourteen years!* There used to be eleven employees and today these five hold down the fort.

Cheryl is a soft spoken, articulate woman with a heart of gold. I barely got in the door when she graciously offered to serve me lunch. As she tried to eat, she also fielded questions from members of the Full Circle Community. She was getting ready to serve people that wanted seconds and kept track of the ones who arrived late and needed to be first in the line since they missed the first serving! She has mastered the art of multi-tasking. Her degree in Psychology along with her management skills would be highly valued in a much higher paying position. I am so thankful for her loving heart that is willing to be there for Kim and the others.

I felt a sense of urgency after meeting with Cheryl. Further research revealed a *national disgrace that nobody seems to talk about*. There are literally hundreds of small towns like Ypsilanti in every state, but the vast majority don't have any place like Full Circle for people with a mental health condition.

While I am extremely grateful for Kim's ideal situation with the incredible support she receives in our small community, I am deeply disturbed with the realization that millions of people with a mental health condition don't have this assistance. It is a national deficit that needs our attention!

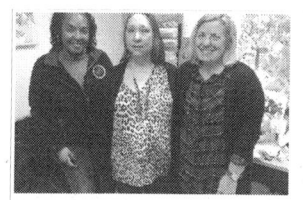
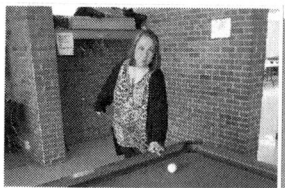

Case Manager Angela Donald & Psychiatric Nurse Practitioner Sharon Stetz surround Kim with constant support.

Kim enjoys the pool table at Full Circle Community Center. This "home away from home" is wonderful incentive to stay involved instead of isolating.

When I asked Cheryl what she would like to see implemented at Full Circle to improve it, I was shocked at her response. "I would love to see the students from the University of Michigan return. They used to come and receive credit for their contribution to our members, but they now are assigned "virtual patients." Kim's favorite time of year is in the Fall when Eastern Michigan University students come to her apartment complex and do arts and crafts with the residents and facilitate games.

I tried to wrap my brain around this new direction some administrator put in place. No "virtual" patient could ever help students develop more compassion and a genuine understanding of the challenges Kim and others experience daily. But even worse, students bring a positive youthful energy to the members of Full Circle. They are now deprived of this dynamic energy which helps them engage with people who do not have mental illness.

Our mentally ill used to be shut away in large institutions. Today their support programs are often the first thing to lose funding when budgets are cut.

Our community center citizens have now been replaced by "virtual" patients for college students. *What does this say about our national conscience?*

People with a mental health condition strike a deep nerve of fear within society because they make us realize how fragile our lives are when the brain is the organ that is ill. It's easier to look away and try not to notice their plight. But there are thousands of families that do not have that option when their loved one becomes ill.

Five public servants keep our community center active. I can only imagine how tired they must be at the end of each week after feeding and caring for so many people. It is a labor of love and hopefully this love will be rewarded with the funding needed to maintain our Center for many more years.

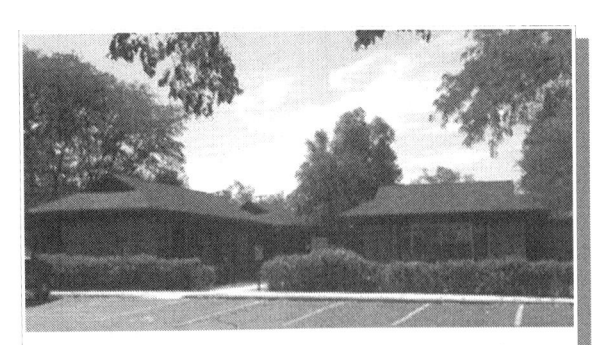

Full Circle Community Center is a "home away from home" for our mentally ill citizens.

# Kim's gift to us all

At the time of this writing, Kim is 45 years old and her most enduring trait is her gratitude for everything she has been blessed with in life. I cannot remember a time when she complained or even felt sorry for herself. She finds enjoyment from the simplest things in her day.

She is stable with medications the doctors monitor closely. She is surrounded by friends, family, and a community support team that consists of a case manager, psychiatrist, and the Full Circle Community support staff. Churches occasionally send volunteers to her apartment complex and provide entertainment for the residents. Eastern Michigan University students come every autumn to play jeopardy, karaoke, and do craft projects. They bring food and wonderful positive energy to the residents.

*She is content.* That is what every parent wishes for a child: to be happy and content with life, despite its many challenges.

Her current challenge is blocking out the voices to get dressed each day. I asked her why she had to get up at 5 am when she had an 8 am doctor appointment. The voices command her to change her clothes over and over for an hour or more! Making out her grocery list is also a big accomplishment as the voices demand she start over again and again.

Stuttering when her brain races makes communication frustrating at times. She trains herself to speak very slowly when this occurs which requires great mental discipline.

Her weight gain had made life much more difficult. Seat belts did not fit anymore, and this was a huge wakeup call because she enjoys getting out of the apartment to shop. We devised a plan that enabled her to lose 65 pounds through eating Weight Watchers meals. That is a huge accomplishment for anyone, especially someone with mental illness.

Short term memory has also deteriorated significantly. As her social security payee representative, I bring her the money she needs for groceries and laundry each month. It is exactly the same every month, but I will receive at least four or five calls reminding me what I need to bring.

The calls begin with, "Hi, Mom, can you bring my money this week? I need my spending money in $1's and $5's. And don't forget my quarters for the laundry."

"I am bringing it tomorrow," I respond patiently.

A few hours later, "Mom, I need my money for this month."

"I know sweetie. I told you I have it ready."

"Oh, I forgot. OK!"

Thirty minutes later the caller ID says "Kim" and I know exactly what she will say.

"Hi Mom. When are you bringing my money?"

"Don't you remember I just told you I will be there tomorrow."

"Oh, I forgot. Sorry to bother you."

There are days when five calls are ten minutes apart. Eventually I turn off my ringer and have learned not to feel guilty about it. This is when I must dig deep for love that is patient. Even the most patient caregivers can find their spiritual resources stretched to their limit. I remind myself to be grateful she is so happy in spite of her many challenges.

Some schizophrenics develop dementia or Alzheimer's as they age. Since the future is not predictable, there is one thing I know I can always depend on. *Faith, hope and love* will sustain us no matter what each day brings.

When I considered sharing Kim's story, I thought the world didn't need another book. I wrote it anyway because just like the boy who continued to toss one more star fish in the sea, perhaps our story will make a difference in your life.

If Kim's story inspires you, pause for a moment and *feel deep gratitude for life*. Think about *the simple everyday things* that make up 90% of your life. It's tempting to let problems overshadow all the good which surrounds us. No matter what the challenge is, you too can rely on *faith, hope and love* to strengthen and support you.

Kim is my role model through her *uncommon courage*. She continues to find something to be grateful for in her daily life, despite her many challenges. She refuses to allow the "voices" of schizophrenia to drown out her own thoughts which bring her peace and joy. She has achieved spiritual mastery of Philippians 4:8.

> *Whatever is true, noble, honest,*
> *just, lovely, commendable,*
> *excellent and worthy of praise,*
> *think on these things.*

# Epilogue: It is well with my soul

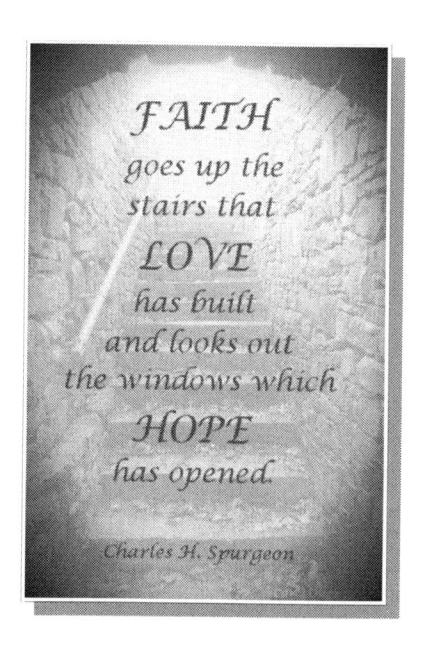

FAITH goes up the stairs that LOVE has built and looks out the windows which HOPE has opened.

*Charles H. Spurgeon*

As I become aware that I am in the final chapter of my own life, I think about the spiritual gifts I have received. Those who have stayed faithful to their religious beliefs for a lifetime might view my story as unstable, one with far too much diversity.

I have been a Lutheran, Baptist, Methodist, and Mormon. I was the World Missions Director for a non-denominational church in New Braunfels,

Texas. I was a Christian missionary in Mexico for twelve years. I was the Administrative Director for a Unity church in Farmington Hills, Michigan. I have read books by authors from every spiritual persuasion.

I spent most of my life hoping to discover how to really *know* this Creator we call God. I finally discovered what this Creator *wanted me to know*. God isn't very interested in our doctrines. There are millions of people from every walk of life who have received miracles and commune daily with our Creator.

Love is foremost in the Divine Mind! I don't mean the emotion we experience that we call "love." Love is the divine energy or spirit that creates, sustains, supports and maintains every life form in the universe. It always expands, deepens and increases us, never diminishing or tearing us down. Love works behind the veil of our consciousness to bring something helpful and good out of *every situation*.

It's easy to know when we are aligned with this Holy Spirit of love. Any thought, word or deed that tears someone down or diminishes them is out of alignment with this love. This is the root cause of all our suffering.

My greatest anxiety as I entered my sixties was what would happen to Kim if I passed away before she did. But that fear has finally disappeared. I now know that the love I have for her is the very Spirit of God, which I have been privileged to experience as her Mother.

Love is eternal, dependable and trustworthy. Love permeates the entire universe. "It causes me to lay down in green pastures and It restores my soul. It fears no evil." I can trust this amazing Love to watch over my precious Kim even if it is not through me.

**_It is well with my soul._**

# Acknowledgments

Special thanks to John Skroder for your meticulous editing and encouragement.

Much appreciation to friends and family who gave me encouragement and help with memories.

Rachele Doray, George Karlsven, Elaine Koehler, Barb Donn, Marsha Scherbel, Debbie Hassett -Stolz, Tammy Erlanson, and Emilie Lin: your support made this project possible.

42027467R00060

Made in the USA
Middletown, DE
10 April 2019